Atkins Diet Cookbook 2024

100 Tasty And Easy Low-Carb Recipes for Wellness And Weight-loss

By Sharon Byers

Disclaimer

The information contained in this book is for general informational purposes only. The author and publisher make no representation or warranties of any kind, express or implied, about the completeness, accuracy, reliability, suitability, or availability with respect to the information, products, services, or related graphics contained in this book for any purpose. Any reliance you place on such information is therefore strictly at your own risk.

In no event will the author or publisher be liable for any loss or damage including without limitation, indirect or consequential loss or damage, or any loss or damage whatsoever arising from loss of data or profits arising out of, or in connection with, the use of this book.

While every effort has been made to ensure that the information in this book is accurate and up-to-date, the author and publisher do not warrant that the information will be kept up-to-date, be true, accurate, complete, or non-misleading.

Any views or opinions represented in this book are personal and belong solely to the author and do not represent those of people, institutions, or organizations that the author may or may not be associated with in professional or personal capacity unless explicitly stated.

TABLE OF CONTENTS

Introduction To The Atkins Diet

The Atkins Diet is a low-carbohydrate diet designed to promote weight loss and improve overall health. The Atkins Diet, which was introduced in the early 1970s, has undergone various modifications over the years, turning into a popular nutritional regimen that has drawn both praise and criticism. This overview aims to provide an overview of the Atkins Diet, its concepts, stages, potential benefits and concerns for those considering following this eating plan.

The Atkins Diet's Foundations:

The Atkins Diet is based on the idea that lowering carbohydrate intake can result in significant weight loss and improved health. Unlike traditional low-fat diets that limit calorie intake, the Atkins Diet focuses on lowering carbs, the body's primary source of energy. By reducing carbohydrate ingestion, the body enters ketosis, a state in which it burns fat for fuel rather than glucose produced by carbs.

The Atkins Diet is divided into four stages, each of which serves a specific purpose in the weight loss process.

1. Induction Phase:

   - Goal: Enter ketosis and begin losing weight.

   - Duration: 2 weeks on average.

   - Carbohydrate Intake: 20-25 grams per day, mostly from vegetables.

   - Foods: Meat, fish, eggs and leafy greens are examples of high-fat, moderate-protein, low-carb foods.

2. Balancing Phase(OWL - Ongoing Weight Loss)

   - Goal: Reintroduce more carbohydrates gradually while maintaining weight loss.

   - Duration: 10 pounds less than desired weight.

   - Carbohydrate consumption: Increase carbohydrate consumption weekly in small increments, focusing on nutrient-dense carbohydrates.

   - Foods: Increasing dietary options by including nuts, seeds and low-carb fruits.

3. Pre-Maintenance Phase: - ideal: Get closer to your ideal weight and fine-tune your carb tolerance.

- Duration: As weight loss slows, it can take months.

- Carbohydrate Intake: Continued gradual increase based on individual response.

- Foods: Increased the amount of starchy vegetables and grains.

4. Maintenance Phase: - Goal: Maintain weight loss and promote long-term health.

- Indefinite duration.

- Carbohydrate intake: Maintain carbohydrate intake at a level that maintains weight without growing.

- Foods: Maintain a balanced and consistent low-carb eating habit.

Principles of the Atkins Diet:

1. Carbohydrate Restriction: The cornerstone of the Atkins Diet is reducing carbohydrate consumption to generate a metabolic condition called ketosis. By doing so, the body changes from burning glucose to burning stored fat for energy.

2. Protein Intake: Adequate protein consumption is suggested to assist muscle maintenance and prevent muscle loss during weight loss. Protein-rich meals like meat, fish and eggs are mainstays in the Atkins Diet.

3. Healthy Fats: Contrary to the low-fat tendency of many diets, the Atkins Diet promotes healthy fats. Avocados, nuts, seeds and olive oil are suggested to offer vital fatty acids and satiety.

4. Phased Approach: The diet is divided into phases to assist gradual adjustment to varying levels of carbohydrate consumption. This staged method seeks to avoid quick weight return and encourage long-term success.

5. Individualization: The Atkins Diet understands that individuals have varying sensitivities to carbs. It highlights the need of establishing a carb consumption amount that is sustainable and effective for each person.

Potential Benefits of the Atkins Diet:

1. Weight reduction: One of the key reasons individuals adopt the Atkins Diet is its effectiveness in facilitating weight reduction. By limiting carb consumption, the body changes

into a state of ketosis, leading to enhanced fat burning and, eventually, weight reduction.

2. Blood Sugar Control: The Atkins Diet may benefit persons with type 2 diabetes by helping manage blood sugar levels. The reduction in carbohydrate consumption can lead to enhanced insulin sensitivity and better glycemic management.

3. Appetite Suppression: High-protein and high-fat diets can create a sensation of fullness, lowering overall calorie consumption. This can be particularly effective for people wanting to regulate their appetite and decrease cravings.

4. Improved Lipid Profile: Some research show that the Atkins Diet may positively influence lipid profiles by raising high-density lipoprotein (HDL) cholesterol and lowering triglyceride levels.

5. Enhanced Mental Clarity: Advocates of low-carb diets, particularly the Atkins Diet, generally report greater mental clarity and focus. This is linked to the steady blood sugar levels attained by reduced carb consumption.

Considerations and Criticisms:

While the Atkins Diet has gained popularity, it has also received criticism and concerns. Some considerations include:

1. Nutritional Intake: The limitation of some food categories, notably fruits and whole grains in the first phases, may lead to possible nutritional deficits. Individuals should ensure they acquire vital vitamins and minerals through food choices or supplementation.

2. Sustainability: Critics believe that the restricted aspect of the Atkins Diet, especially in the induction period, may be tough to continue over the long run. Sustainable dietary adjustments are key for sustained health effects.

3. Potential Health dangers: There are worries regarding the potential health dangers linked with a diet heavy in saturated fats, such as those found in red meat. Individuals with particular health disorders, such as cardiovascular difficulties, should contact with healthcare specialists before following the Atkins Diet.

4. Individual Responses: Not everyone responds the same way to low-carb diets. Individual factors, including genetics

and metabolic rate, can alter the success and safety of the Atkins Diet for an individual person.

The Atkins Diet, with its emphasis on carbohydrate restriction and phased approach, has had a key impact in redefining dietary ideas. While it has shown promise in aiding weight reduction and controlling some health concerns, consumers should approach it with great thought. Consulting with healthcare providers, monitoring nutrient consumption and customizing the diet to individual needs are critical steps for anyone contemplating the Atkins Diet. As with any dietary plan, balance, sustainability and long-term health should stay at the center of one's nutritional decisions.

Understanding The Atkins Diet Phases

A Comprehensive Overview

The Atkins Diet is separated into four stages because of its low-carbohydrate approach to weight loss and greater health. Each phase has a specific purpose, guiding people through a gradual process of carbohydrate reintroduction, weight loss and maintenance. We go into the nuances of each phase, revealing their goals, dietary restrictions, potential issues and overall contributions to the success of the Atkins Diet in this in-depth investigation.

1. Ketosis Initiation and Rapid Weight Loss Objectives: The Atkins Diet begins with the Induction Phase. Its primary objectives are to promote rapid weight loss and to induce ketosis, a metabolic state in which the body burns stored fat for energy. This two-week phase establishes the foundation for the diet's subsequent stages.

Dietary Recommendations: - Limit carbohydrate consumption to 20-25 grams per day, primarily from non-starchy veggies.

- Meals: High-fat, moderate-protein, low-carb meals include meat, fish, eggs and leafy greens.

- Nutrient Considerations: During the initial restricted phase, individuals are encouraged to consume nutrient-dense foods in order to compensate for any deficiencies.

- Carbohydrate Withdrawal: As the body adjusts to reduced carbohydrate intake, some people may experience carbohydrate withdrawal symptoms such as fatigue, headaches and irritability.

- Ketosis adaptation: Achieving and maintaining ketosis can be difficult and some people may require several days to adjust adequately.

- Rapid Weight Loss: The significant decrease in carbohydrate consumption causes rapid water weight loss, which adds to an early decline in overall body weight.

- Appetite control: High-fat, moderate-protein diets help with appetite control by reducing cravings and increasing feelings of fullness.

2. Balancing Phase (OWL - Ongoing Weight Loss): Carbohydrate Reintroduction Gradually.

Following the Induction Phase, the Balancing Phase attempts to gradually reintroduce more carbs while maintaining weight loss progress. The emphasis shifts away from fast weight loss and toward a more maintained and controlled technique.

Dietary Recommendations: - Carbohydrate intake: Weekly carbohydrate consumption should be increased, with a focus on nutrient-dense carbs.

- Foods: Nuts, seeds and low-carb fruits are examples of foods that promote nutritional diversity.

- Nutrient Factors to Consider: Continue to prioritize nutrient-dense foods to preserve overall wellness.

- Carb Sensitivity: Individuals may need to assess their carb tolerance before increasing carb consumption, since some meals may have a higher impact on ketosis than others.

- It may be challenging to strike the right balance between reintroducing carbohydrates and maintaining weight loss.

Benefits: - Long-Term Weight Loss: Reintroducing carbohydrates gradually enables for long-term weight loss while expanding meal options.

- Individualized Approach: Enables users to modify their carb consumption based on their responses and preferences.

3. Pre-Maintenance Phase: Approaching Your Goal Weight and Fine-Tuning

The Pre-Maintenance Phase focuses on fine-tuning carbohydrate tolerance and preparing individuals for the Maintenance Phase once they have reached their goal weight. The nutritional plan is being fine-tuned for long-term success.

- Carbohydrate Intake: Continued gradual increase based on individual reaction and weight loss results.

- Foods: Increased consumption of starchy vegetables and grains, resulting in a more balanced diet.

- Weight loss plateau: Some people may have a weight loss plateau during this time, prompting dietary changes.

- Long-Term Dedication: The issue is maintaining the discipline and dedication required for long-term weight loss.

Individuals can modify their approach to carb consumption based on their individual sensitivities, resulting in a sustainable and personalized diet.

- Maintenance Preparation: Lays the framework for transitioning to the Maintenance Phase with a firm understanding of one's nutritional requirements.

4. Long-Term Weight Loss and Health Maintenance

The Atkins Diet's third step, the Maintenance step, focuses on maintaining weight loss and promoting long-term health. It requires sticking to a well-balanced and long-term low-carb diet.

Dietary Recommendations: - Carbohydrate intake: Keep carbohydrate intake at a level that allows you to maintain your weight without gaining weight.

- Foods: A well-balanced and diverse diet rich in nutrient-dense foods is emphasized.

- Dietary Adherence: The issue is keeping a low-carb diet on a consistent basis, because some people may struggle with the absence of some high-carb items.

- Weight Maintenance: Maintaining weight loss can be tough because it requires a consistent commitment to healthy eating habits.

- Sustained Weight Loss: Provides a foundation for maintaining weight loss achieved during the first phases of the Atkins Diet.

- Long-Term Health: Encourages a healthy and sustainable diet, which may increase general well-being.

Considerations and Modifications:

1. Individual reactions: The Atkins Diet recognizes that individual carbohydrate consumption reactions vary. It promotes self-monitoring and changes depending on personal progress.

2. Nutrient Intake: Nutrient intake must be monitored at all stages. Individuals should make sure they get enough vitamins and minerals through food or supplementation.

3. Physical exercise: Regular physical exercise is essential for the success of the Atkins Diet. Exercise complements a healthy diet by improving overall health and well-being.

4. Hydration: Adequate hydration is stressed throughout the process to assist various biological activities such as digestion and metabolism.

Getting the Most Out of the Atkins Diet Phases

The planned progression through the phases of the Atkins Diet offers individuals with a method for achieving and maintaining weight loss while also improving overall health. Individuals can better meet their nutritional demands and make educated decisions when they are aware of the particular objectives, dietary recommendations and possible obstacles linked with each stage.

While the Atkins Diet has proven to be useful in terms of weight loss and managing specific health concerns for many people, it is crucial to approach it holistically. The Atkins Diet's overall efficacy is highly dependent on individual sensitivities, sustainability over the long term and dedication to healthy lifestyle behaviors.

People with pre-existing health conditions should seek the advice of healthcare professionals, registered dietitians, or nutritionists before beginning any new diet program. The Atkins Diet has the potential to be an effective tool in the fight for and preservation of a healthy weight and way of life when used with purpose and a focus on the long term.

A Comprehensive Guide To Atkins Cooking Ingredients

The Atkins Diet, recognized for its low-carbohydrate approach, stresses a specific set of nutrients to achieve its nutritional goals. Whether you're a seasoned Atkins dieter or new to this dietary paradigm, learning the fundamentals is essential for making delicious and satisfying meals while adhering to the diet's principles. In this extensive guide, we delve into the key components that form the foundation of Atkins cuisine, providing insights into their roles, variations and how they contribute to a good low-carb culinary experience.

1. Proteins: The Building Blocks of Atkins Meals

Proteins are the foundation of the Atkins Diet, aiding in the satisfaction of hunger, the improvement of muscular performance and the general satiety. Here are several essential protein sources included in Atkins cooking:

a. Meat: - Variety: Meats such as beef, pork, lamb, fowl (chicken, turkey) and game meats are available.

- Cuts: Choose lean cuts to limit your saturated fat consumption. Examples include sirloin, tenderloin and skinless poultry.

b. Seafood and Fish: - Fatty Fish: Omega-3 fatty acids are abundant in fatty fish such as salmon, mackerel and sardines.

- White fish such as cod, haddock and flounder are high in protein but low in fat.

c. Eggs: - Flexibility: Eggs are a versatile and low-cost protein source that can be employed in a variety of Atkins recipes.

- Omega-3 enhanced: Use omega-3 enhanced eggs for added nutritional benefit.

d. Dairy products: - Cheese: Use cheeses like cheddar, mozzarella and feta in moderation for flavor and richness.

- Greek Yogurt: Use full-fat, unsweetened Greek yogurt for a protein-rich, low-carb snack.

e. Proteins derived from plants: - Tofu and Tempeh: These soy-based proteins are good for Atkins vegetarians and add variety to recipes.

- Edamame (edamame): Edamame, which is high in protein and low in carbs, is a great addition to salads and stir-fries.

Cooking Tip: - Grilling and Roasting: By grilling or roasting meats, fish and fowl, you can enhance their flavor. The Maillard process adds depth and richness to dishes without relying on high-carb ingredients.

2. Healthy Fats as Fuel for Your Low-Carb Journey

While the Atkins Diet limits carbohydrate intake, it encourages the consumption of healthy fats. These fats are an important source of energy and contribute to a feeling of fullness. For Atkins cooking, the following healthy fats are required:

a. Avocado: - Versatility: Avocado gives recipes a creamy smoothness while also delivering a nutrient-dense source of beneficial monounsaturated fats.

- Guacamole: To make a filling dip, mash avocados with lime juice, garlic and seasonings.

b. Extra Virgin Olive Oil: Extra virgin olive oil is preferred for its rich flavor and antioxidant properties.

- Salad Dressings: To prepare low-carb salad dressings, use olive oil, vinegar and herbs.

Medium-Chain Triglycerides (MCTs): MCTs are a type of fat that is swiftly converted into energy and are found in coconut oil.

- Cooking and Baking: High-heat cooking and low-carb baking are both possible.

d. Walnuts, Almonds and Pecans These healthful fat-rich almonds make substantial snacks or salad toppings.

- Chia and Flax Seeds: Chia seeds and flaxseeds are abundant in omega-3 fatty acids and work well in smoothies and low-carb baked goods.

f. Butter and ghee:

- Ghee (clarified butter): A lactose-free replacement with a high smoke point, ghee is ideal for cooking.

Cooking Tip: - Flavor Infusion: Infuse oils with herbs and spices to give depth and richness to your recipes without relying on high-carb sauces.

3. Nutritious and flavorful Vegetables with Low Carbohydrates

Atkins promotes low-carb vegetables, which provide vital nutrients, fiber and a variety of flavors. Here are some vegetables that are suitable for the Atkins diet:

a. Leafy Greens: Spinach, Kale and Swiss Chard are high in vitamins and minerals and can be used to make salads and side dishes.

Cruciferous vegetables include broccoli, cauliflower and Brussels sprouts. These low-carb vegetables can be roasted, sautéed, or added to low-carb casseroles.

c. Eggplant and Zucchini: - Carbohydrate Substitutes: Zucchini noodles (zoodles) and eggplant slices are excellent low-carb substitutes for traditional pasta and lasagna sheets.

d. Tomatoes and bell peppers: - Moderation: While bell peppers and tomatoes contain more carbohydrates than leafy greens, they can be included in moderation for flavor.

e. Green Beans with Asparagus: - Roasting and Sautéing: Roast asparagus or sauté green beans with garlic and olive oil for a delicious side meal.

Grilling vegetables imparts a smokey flavor while boosting their natural sweetness without the use of high-carb spices.

4. Low-Carb Flours and Substitutes: Carb-Free Baking

For those who enjoy baking, low-carb flours and replacements allow them to create tasty treats without violating the Atkins Diet's principles. Low-carb baking necessitates the following ingredients:

a. Nutrient-Dense Almond Flour: Almond flour is a low-carb, high-nutrient alternative to wheat flour.

- Baking: You may use almond flour to make low-carb bread, muffins and pancakes.

b. Coconut Flour: - Absorbency: Coconut flour absorbs more liquid than almond flour, requiring recipe modifications.

- Gluten-Free: Ideal for those following the gluten-free Atkins diet.

c. Flaxseed Meal: - Omega-3 Fatty Acids: Flaxseeds provide omega-3 fatty acids to baked goods.

- Egg Substitute: Make a plant-based egg substitute by combining flaxseed meal and water.

d. Powdered Psyllium Husk: - Texture Enhancement: Psyllium husk powder adds structure and moisture to low-carb baked goods.

- Keto-friendly Bread: This ingredient is used to improve the texture of keto-friendly bread recipes.

Stevia, Erythritol and Monk Fruit are sugar substitutes that provide sweetness without boosting blood sugar levels.

- Baking and cooking: It can be used to sweeten desserts, sauces and beverages.

Flours Blending: Combining almond flour with coconut flour or flaxseed meal results in a balanced texture in baked goods.

5. Flavor Enhancers: spices, herbs and condiments

Maintaining a low-carb diet does not require giving up flavor. Herbs, spices and condiments provide richness and diversity to Atkins dishes:

a. Herbs: Basil, Thyme, Rosemary and Oregano: Fresh or dried herbs enhance the flavor of dishes.

- Infused with herbs Oils: Infuse olive oil with herbs to give flavor to your dishes.

Cumin, paprika and turmeric are spices that provide warmth and depth to low-carb meals.

- Homemade spice blends: Create your own spice blends to season meats and vegetables with.

c. Garlic and ginger:

- Fresh and Ground: Fresh and ground garlic and ginger add fragrant richness.

- Stir-Fries and Sauces: Essential for Asian-inspired dishes and low-carb sauces.

d. Condiments: Mustard, Vinegar and Hot Sauce: These low-carb condiments add tang and taste without adding sugar.

Richness is added to a number of recipes by using full-fat mayonnaise and sour cream.

c. Zest of lemon, lime and orange: Zest adds brightness and flavor to both sweet and savory dishes.

Experimenting with Flavors: Don't be scared to try new herbs and spices to find taste combinations that appeal to you.

6. Dairy and Cheese: calcium and creaminess

Dairy and cheese products supplement Atkins meals with calcium, protein and richness. Moderation is crucial, however, because some dairy products may contain hidden sugars. Choose full-fat alternatives wherever possible:

a. Cheddars: For a great finishing touch, grate or melt Cheddar, Mozzarella and Parmesan.

- Cream cheese: Adds creaminess to both sweet and savory meals.

b. Whole Milk: - Creaminess: Creaminess is added to sauces, soups and desserts by using heavy cream.

- Whipping Cream: Whip up some whipping cream for a low-carb dessert or coffee topper.

c. Cooking and Baking: Sautéing, baking and adding richness to dishes are all wonderful uses for butter and ghee.

d. Cottage Cheese: - High Protein: Choose full-fat cottage cheese for a protein-rich snack or ingredient in recipes.

Cream of Tartar:

- Toppings: Add to low-carb meals as a final touch.

- Creamy Dressings: Add to salad dressings or dips to make a creamy dressing.

Melted cheeses add a nice and creamy touch to a variety of low-carb meals, from casseroles to omelets.

To navigate the world of Atkins cuisine, careful ingredient selection that corresponds to the diet's guidelines is required. Balance and diversity are essential when preparing a protein-rich meal, experimenting with low-carb flours, or enhancing flavors with herbs and spices.

By including these essential ingredients into your Atkins culinary arsenal, you will not only meet the program's nutritional requirements, but you will also be able to prepare tasty, satisfying meals that will benefit your overall health. Remember to personalize your Atkins journey by trying new meals and cuisines to discover a low-carb diet that is both maintainable and enjoyable. As with any dietary regimen, consultation with healthcare practitioners or certified dietitians is recommended, especially for people with specific health concerns.

Enjoy the versatility of Atkins cooking in your home while providing your body with nutritious, low-carb pleasures.

BREAKFAST

1. Keto Bacon and Egg Cups:

Ingredients:

- Eggs

- Bacon strips

- Salt and pepper (to taste)

- Chopped fresh chives (optional for garnish)

Instructions:

1. Preheat the oven to 375°F (190°C).

2. Line muffin tin cups with bacon strips, creating a cup shape.

3. Break an egg into each bacon cup.

4. Season with salt and pepper.

5. Bake for 15-20 minutes or until eggs reach desired doneness.

6. Garnish with chopped chives if desired.

Prep Time: 25 minutes

2. Spinach and Feta Omelet:

Ingredients:

- Eggs

- Fresh spinach leaves

- Feta cheese, crumbled

- Salt and pepper (to taste)

- Olive oil or butter for cooking

Instructions:

1. Beat the eggs in a bowl and season with salt and pepper.

2. Heat olive oil or butter in a pan over medium heat.

3. Add fresh spinach and cook until wilted.

4. Pour the beaten eggs over the spinach.

5. Sprinkle crumbled feta cheese on top.

6. Cook until the edges set, then fold the omelet in half.

7. Cook until the center is done.

Prep Time: 15 minutes

3. Almond Flour Pancakes:

Ingredients:

- Almond flour

- Eggs

- Unsweetened almond milk

- Baking powder

- Vanilla extract

- Salt

- Butter or coconut oil (for cooking)

Instructions:

1. In a bowl, whisk together almond flour, eggs, almond milk, baking powder, vanilla extract and a pinch of salt.

2. Heat butter or coconut oil in a pan over medium heat.

3. Pour batter onto the pan to form pancakes.

4. Cook until bubbles form on the surface, then flip and cook the other side.

5. Repeat with the remaining batter.

Prep Time: 20 minutes

4. Avocado and Bacon Breakfast Wrap:

Ingredients:

- Large lettuce leaves (as wraps)

- Avocado, sliced

- Cooked bacon strips

- Scrambled eggs

- Salsa (optional)

- Salt and pepper (to taste)

Instructions:

1. Lay lettuce leaves flat.

2. Spread sliced avocado on each leaf.

3. Add cooked bacon strips and scrambled eggs.

4. Season with salt and pepper.

5. Optionally, add salsa for extra flavor.

6. Wrap and enjoy.

Prep Time: 15 minutes

5. Keto Chia Seed Pudding:

Ingredients:

- Chia seeds

- Unsweetened almond milk

- Vanilla extract

- Stevia or sweetener of choice

- Berries (for topping)

Instructions:

1. Mix chia seeds, almond milk, vanilla extract and sweetener in a bowl.

2. Stir well and let it sit for 5 minutes.

3. Stir again and refrigerate for at least 2 hours or overnight.

4. Top with fresh berries before serving.

Prep Time: 5 minutes (plus chilling time)

6. Smoked Salmon and Cream Cheese Roll-ups:

Ingredients:

- Smoked salmon slices

- Cream cheese

- Fresh dill (optional)

- Lemon wedges (for serving)

Instructions:

1. Lay smoked salmon slices flat.

2. Spread a layer of cream cheese on each slice.

3. Optionally, sprinkle fresh dill over the cream cheese.

4. Roll up the smoked salmon slices.

5. Serve with lemon wedges.

Prep Time: 10 minutes

7. Sausage and Veggie Breakfast Casserole:

Ingredients:

- Sausage, cooked and crumbled

- Bell peppers, diced

- Onion, diced

- Eggs

- Heavy cream

- Shredded cheese

- Salt and pepper (to taste)

Instructions:

1. Preheat the oven to 375°F (190°C).

2. In a greased baking dish, spread cooked sausage, bell peppers and onions.

3. In a bowl, whisk eggs, heavy cream, salt and pepper together.

4. Pour the egg mixture over the sausage and veggies.

5. Sprinkle shredded cheese on top.

6. Bake for 25-30 minutes or until the center is set.

Prep Time: 30 minutes

8. Low-Carb Breakfast Burrito Bowl:

Ingredients:

- Cauliflower rice

- Ground breakfast sausage

- Eggs, scrambled

- Avocado, sliced

- Salsa

- Shredded cheese

- Salt and pepper (to taste)

Instructions:

1. Cook cauliflower rice according to package instructions.

2. In a pan, cook ground sausage until browned.

3. Scramble eggs in the same pan.

4. Assemble bowls with cauliflower rice, sausage, scrambled eggs, sliced avocado, salsa and shredded cheese.

5. Season with salt and pepper.

Prep Time: 25 minutes

9. Greek Yogurt Parfait with Berries:

Ingredients:

- Greek yogurt (unsweetened)

- Berries (strawberries, blueberries, raspberries)

- Almonds, chopped

- Unsweetened coconut flakes

- Stevia or sweetener of choice (optional)

Instructions:

1. Layer Greek yogurt in a glass or bowl.

2. Add a layer of mixed berries.

3. Sprinkle chopped almonds and coconut flakes on top.

4. Optionally, sweeten with stevia.

5. Repeat layers and finish with berries on top.

Prep Time: 10 minutes

10. Keto Egg Muffins with Ham and Cheese:

Ingredients:

- Eggs

- Ham, diced

- Shredded cheese

- Bell peppers, diced

- Salt and pepper (to taste)

- Chopped chives (optional for garnish)

Instructions:

1. Preheat the oven to 375°F (190°C).

2. In a bowl, whisk together eggs, diced ham, shredded cheese, diced bell peppers, salt and pepper.

3. Pour the mixture into greased muffin cups.

4. Bake for 15-20 minutes or until the muffins are set.

5. Garnish with chopped chives if desired.

Prep Time: 25 minutes

11. Coconut Flour Waffles:

Ingredients:

- Coconut flour

- Eggs

- Almond milk (unsweetened)

- Baking powder

- Vanilla extract

- Stevia or sweetener of choice

- Butter or coconut oil (for cooking)

Instructions:

1. In a bowl, whisk together coconut flour, eggs, almond milk, baking powder, vanilla extract and sweetener.

2. Let the batter rest for a few minutes.

3. Preheat a waffle iron and grease with butter or coconut oil.

4. Pour batter onto the iron and cook according to the waffle iron instructions.

5. Serve with your favorite low-carb toppings.

Prep Time: 15 minutes

12. Zucchini and Cheese Frittata:

Ingredients:

- Eggs

- Zucchini, grated

- Cheddar cheese, shredded

- Onion, diced

- Salt and pepper (to taste)

- Olive oil or butter for cooking

Instructions:

1. Preheat the oven to 375°F (190°C).

2. In an oven-safe skillet, sauté diced onions in olive oil or butter until softened.

3. Add grated zucchini and cook until excess moisture evaporates.

4. In a bowl, whisk eggs, salt and pepper. Pour over the vegetables.

5. Sprinkle shredded cheddar cheese on top.

6. Cook on the stovetop for a few minutes, then transfer to the oven and bake until set.

7. Slice and serve.

Prep Time: 25 minutes

13. Keto Avocado Toast with Poached Eggs:

Ingredients:

- Avocado

- Eggs

- Almond flour bread or low-carb bread alternative

- Lemon juice

- Salt and pepper (to taste)

- Red pepper flakes (optional for spice)

Instructions:

1. Toast almond flour bread or a low-carb bread alternative.

2. Mash avocado and spread it over the toasted bread.

3. Poach eggs and place them on top of the mashed avocado.

4. Squeeze lemon juice over the eggs and season with salt, pepper and red pepper flakes if desired.

Prep Time: 15 minutes

14. Mushroom and Bacon Egg Bake:

Ingredients:

- Eggs

- Mushrooms, sliced

- Bacon, cooked and crumbled

- Shredded cheese

- Green onions, chopped

- Salt and pepper (to taste)

- Butter for greasing

Instructions:

1. Preheat the oven to 375°F (190°C).

2. Grease a baking dish with butter.

3. Crack eggs into the dish and whisk.

4. Add sliced mushrooms, crumbled bacon, shredded cheese and chopped green onions.

5. Season with salt and pepper.

6. Bake until the eggs are set and the top is golden brown.

Prep Time: 30 minutes

15. Keto Breakfast Pizza:

Ingredients:

- Almond flour crust (pre-made or homemade)

- Cream cheese

- Eggs

- Bacon, cooked and crumbled

- Shredded mozzarella cheese

- Cherry tomatoes, sliced

- Fresh basil leaves

- Salt and pepper (to taste)

Instructions:

1. Preheat the oven according to the almond flour crust instructions.

2. Spread a layer of cream cheese over the crust.

3. Crack eggs onto the crust, distributing evenly.

4. Sprinkle crumbled bacon, shredded mozzarella and sliced cherry tomatoes on top.

5. Bake until the crust is golden and the eggs are cooked.

6. Garnish with fresh basil leaves and season with salt and pepper.

Prep Time: 25 minutes

16. Spinach and Mushroom Scramble:

Ingredients:

- Eggs

- Fresh spinach leaves

- Mushrooms, sliced

- Feta cheese, crumbled

- Salt and pepper (to taste)

- Olive oil or butter for cooking

Instructions:

1. In a bowl, beat the eggs and season with salt and pepper.

2. Heat olive oil or butter in a pan over medium heat.

3. Add sliced mushrooms and cook until softened.

4. Add fresh spinach and cook until wilted.

5. Pour the beaten eggs into the pan and scramble.

6. Sprinkle crumbled feta cheese on top and cook until the eggs are done.

Prep Time: 15 minutes

17. Keto Blueberry Muffins:

Ingredients:

- Almond flour

- Eggs

- Unsweetened almond milk

- Baking powder

- Vanilla extract

- Stevia or sweetener of choice

- Blueberries (fresh or frozen)

Instructions:

1. Preheat the oven to 350°F (175°C).

2. In a bowl, mix almond flour, eggs, almond milk, baking powder, vanilla extract and sweetener.

3. Gently fold in blueberries.

4. Spoon the batter into muffin cups.

5. Bake for 20-25 minutes or until a toothpick comes out clean.

Prep Time: 30 minutes

18. Bacon and Cheese Breakfast Casserole:

Ingredients:

- Eggs

- Bacon, cooked and crumbled

- Shredded cheddar cheese

- Heavy cream

- Green onions, chopped

- Salt and pepper (to taste)

- Butter for greasing

Instructions:

1. Preheat the oven to 375°F (190°C).

2. Grease a baking dish with butter.

3. In a bowl, whisk together eggs, heavy cream, salt and pepper.

4. Spread crumbled bacon, shredded cheddar and chopped green onions in the baking dish.

5. Pour the egg mixture over the ingredients.

6. Bake until the eggs are set and the top is golden brown.

Prep Time: 35 minutes

19. Almond Butter Smoothie Bowl:

Ingredients:

- Almond butter

- Unsweetened almond milk

- Spinach leaves

- Protein powder (low-carb)

- Chia seeds

- Berries (for topping)

- Unsweetened coconut flakes (for topping)

Instructions:

1. In a blender, combine almond butter, almond milk, spinach, protein powder and chia seeds.

2. Blend until smooth.

3. Pour the smoothie into a bowl.

4. Top with fresh berries and coconut flakes.

Prep Time: 10 minutes

20. Keto Sausage and Egg McMuffin:

Ingredients:

- Sausage patties (pre-cooked)

- Eggs

- Cheddar cheese slices

- Almond flour English muffins (pre-made or homemade)

- Butter

- Salt and pepper (to taste)

Instructions:

1. Preheat a skillet over medium heat.

2. Cook sausage patties according to package instructions.

3. In the same skillet, melt butter and crack eggs to make fried eggs.

4. Toast almond flour English muffins and spread butter on each half.

5. Assemble the sandwich with sausage, a fried egg and a slice of cheddar cheese.

6. Season with salt and pepper.

Prep Time: 20 minutes

LUNCH

21. Chicken Caesar Salad with Avocado:

Ingredients:

- Grilled chicken breast, sliced

- Romaine lettuce, chopped

- Cherry tomatoes, halved

- Avocado, sliced

- Parmesan cheese, shaved

- Caesar dressing (low-carb)

- Lemon wedges (optional)

Instructions:

1. In a large bowl, combine chopped romaine lettuce, cherry tomatoes and sliced grilled chicken.

2. Add avocado slices and shaved Parmesan cheese.

3. Drizzle with Caesar dressing and toss gently to coat.

4. Serve with lemon wedges if desired.

Prep Time: 15 minutes

22. Keto Cobb Salad:

Ingredients:

- Mixed salad greens

- Grilled chicken breast, diced

- Bacon, cooked and crumbled

- Avocado, diced

- Hard-boiled eggs, sliced

- Blue cheese, crumbled

- Cherry tomatoes, halved

- Keto-friendly ranch dressing

Instructions:

1. Arrange mixed salad greens on a plate.

2. Top with diced grilled chicken, crumbled bacon, diced avocado, sliced hard-boiled eggs, crumbled blue cheese and cherry tomatoes.

3. Drizzle with keto-friendly ranch dressing.

Prep Time: 20 minutes

23. Turkey and Cheese Lettuce Wraps:

Ingredients:

- Turkey slices

- Swiss cheese slices

- Lettuce leaves (large, for wrapping)

- Mayonnaise

- Mustard

- Pickles (optional)

- Salt and pepper (to taste)

Instructions:

1. Lay lettuce leaves flat.

2. Layer turkey slices and Swiss cheese on each leaf.

3. Add mayonnaise, mustard, pickles, salt and pepper.

4. Roll up the lettuce leaves to form wraps.

Prep Time: 10 minutes

24. Caprese Salad Skewers:

Ingredients:

- Cherry tomatoes

- Fresh mozzarella balls

- Basil leaves

- Balsamic glaze (low-carb)

Instructions:

1. Thread cherry tomatoes, fresh mozzarella balls and basil leaves onto skewers.

2. Arrange the skewers on a serving platter.

3. Drizzle with balsamic glaze before serving.

Prep Time: 15 minutes

25. Avocado Tuna Salad:

Ingredients:

- Canned tuna, drained

- Avocado, diced

- Red onion, finely chopped

- Celery, diced

- Mayonnaise

- Dijon mustard

- Salt and pepper (to taste)

- Lettuce leaves (for serving)

Instructions:

1. In a bowl, combine drained tuna, diced avocado, chopped red onion, diced celery, mayonnaise and Dijon mustard.

2. Mix until well combined.

3. Season with salt and pepper.

4. Serve the tuna salad in lettuce leaves.

Prep Time: 10 minutes

26. Broccoli and Cheddar Soup:

Ingredients:

- Broccoli, chopped

- Chicken or vegetable broth (low-sodium)

- Heavy cream

- Cheddar cheese, shredded

- Onion, diced

- Garlic, minced

- Butter

- Salt and pepper (to taste)

Instructions:

1. In a pot, sauté diced onion and minced garlic in butter until softened.

2. Add chopped broccoli and cook for a few minutes.

3. Pour in chicken or vegetable broth and simmer until broccoli is tender.

4. Blend the soup until smooth.

5. Stir in heavy cream and shredded cheddar cheese.

6. Season with salt and pepper.

Prep Time: 30 minutes

27. Keto Egg Salad Lettuce Wraps:

Ingredients:

- Hard-boiled eggs, chopped

- Mayonnaise

- Dijon mustard

- Celery, finely chopped

- Green onions, sliced

- Lettuce leaves (large, for wrapping)

- Salt and pepper (to taste)

Instructions:

1. In a bowl, combine chopped hard-boiled eggs, mayonnaise, Dijon mustard, chopped celery and sliced green onions.

2. Mix until well combined.

3. Season with salt and pepper.

4. Spoon the egg salad onto lettuce leaves and wrap.

Prep Time: 15 minutes

28. Grilled Chicken Salad with Lemon Vinaigrette:

Ingredients:

- Grilled chicken breast, sliced

- Mixed salad greens

- Cherry tomatoes, halved

- Cucumber, sliced

- Red onion, thinly sliced

- Feta cheese, crumbled

- Lemon vinaigrette dressing (low-carb)

Instructions:

1. Combine mixed salad greens, sliced grilled chicken, halved cherry tomatoes, sliced cucumber, thinly sliced red onion and crumbled feta cheese in a large bowl.

2. Drizzle with lemon vinaigrette dressing and toss gently.

Prep Time: 20 minutes

29. Shrimp and Avocado Salad:

Ingredients:

- Cooked shrimp, peeled and deveined

- Avocado, diced

- Cherry tomatoes, halved

- Cilantro, chopped

- Lime juice

- Olive oil

- Salt and pepper (to taste)

- Mixed salad greens

Instructions:

1. In a bowl, combine cooked shrimp, diced avocado, halved cherry tomatoes and chopped cilantro.

2. Drizzle with lime juice and olive oil.

3. Season with salt and pepper.

4. Serve over a bed of mixed salad greens.

Prep Time: 15 minutes

30. Keto Chicken Club Lettuce Wrap:

Ingredients:

- Grilled chicken breast, sliced

- Bacon, cooked and crumbled

- Tomato, sliced

- Avocado, sliced

- Lettuce leaves (large, for wrapping)

- Mayonnaise

- Salt and pepper (to taste)

Instructions:

1. Lay lettuce leaves flat.

2. Layer sliced grilled chicken, crumbled bacon, sliced tomato and sliced avocado on each leaf.

3. Add mayonnaise, salt and pepper.

4. Roll up the lettuce leaves to form wraps.

Prep Time: 15 minutes

31. Greek Salad with Grilled Chicken:

Ingredients:

- Grilled chicken breast, sliced

- Cucumber, diced

- Cherry tomatoes, halved

- Kalamata olives, pitted

- Feta cheese, crumbled

- Red onion, thinly sliced

- Greek dressing (low-carb)

Instructions:

1. In a large bowl, combine sliced grilled chicken, diced cucumber, halved cherry tomatoes, Kalamata olives, crumbled feta cheese and thinly sliced red onion.

2. Drizzle with low-carb Greek dressing and toss gently.

Prep Time: 20 minutes

32. Cauliflower Fried Rice with Shrimp:

Ingredients:

- Cauliflower rice

- Shrimp, peeled and deveined

- Mixed vegetables (e.g., peas, carrots, green onions)

- Garlic, minced

- Soy sauce (low-sodium)

- Sesame oil

- Eggs, beaten

- Salt and pepper (to taste)

Instructions:

1. In a large pan, sauté minced garlic in sesame oil.

2. Add shrimp and cook until pink.

3. Push shrimp to one side and add beaten eggs to the other side, scrambling them.

4. Mix in cauliflower rice, mixed vegetables and soy sauce.

5. Cook until cauliflower rice is tender.

6. Season with salt and pepper.

Prep Time: 25 minutes

33. Zoodle Alfredo with Chicken:

Ingredients:

- Zucchini noodles (zoodles)

- Cooked chicken breast, sliced

- Heavy cream

- Parmesan cheese, grated

- Garlic, minced

- Butter

- Salt and pepper (to taste)

- Fresh parsley (for garnish)

Instructions:

1. In a pan, melt butter and sauté minced garlic until fragrant.

2. Add heavy cream and grated Parmesan cheese, stirring until melted.

3. Add zucchini noodles and cooked sliced chicken.

4. Cook until zoodles are tender.

5. Season with salt and pepper.

6. Garnish with fresh parsley.

Prep Time: 20 minutes

34. Keto BLT Salad:

Ingredients:

- Romaine lettuce, chopped

- Cherry tomatoes, halved

- Bacon, cooked and crumbled

- Avocado, diced

- Blue cheese, crumbled

- Ranch dressing (low-carb)

Instructions:

1. In a large bowl, combine chopped romaine lettuce, halved cherry tomatoes, crumbled bacon, diced avocado and crumbled blue cheese.

2. Drizzle with low-carb ranch dressing and toss gently.

Prep Time: 15 minutes

35. Egg Drop Soup:

Ingredients:

- Chicken or vegetable broth (low-sodium)

- Eggs, beaten

- Green onions, sliced

- Soy sauce (low-sodium)

- Sesame oil

- Salt and pepper (to taste)

Instructions:

1. In a pot, heat chicken or vegetable broth.

2. Stir in beaten eggs in a steady stream, creating ribbons.

3. Add sliced green onions, soy sauce and sesame oil.

4. Season with salt and pepper.

Prep Time: 10 minutes

36. Avocado Chicken Salad:

Ingredients:

- Cooked chicken breast, shredded

- Avocado, diced

- Cherry tomatoes, halved

- Red onion, finely chopped

- Cilantro, chopped

- Lime juice

- Salt and pepper (to taste)

- Lettuce leaves (for serving)

Instructions:

1. In a bowl, combine shredded cooked chicken, diced avocado, halved cherry tomatoes, finely chopped red onion and chopped cilantro.

2. Drizzle with lime juice and toss gently.

3. Season with salt and pepper.

4. Serve in lettuce leaves.

Prep Time: 15 minutes

37. Spinach and Bacon Salad:

Ingredients:

- Baby spinach leaves

- Bacon, cooked and crumbled

- Hard-boiled eggs, sliced

- Mushrooms, sliced

- Red onion, thinly sliced

- Keto-friendly vinaigrette dressing

Instructions:

1. In a large bowl, combine baby spinach leaves, crumbled bacon, sliced hard-boiled eggs, sliced mushrooms and thinly sliced red onion.

2. Drizzle with keto-friendly vinaigrette dressing and toss gently.

Prep Time: 15 minutes

38. Cauliflower Crust Pizza:

Ingredients:

- Cauliflower crust (pre-made or homemade)

- Sugar-free pizza sauce

- Mozzarella cheese, shredded

- Toppings of choice (e.g., pepperoni, olives, bell peppers)

- Italian seasoning

- Olive oil

Instructions:

1. Preheat the oven according to the cauliflower crust instructions.

2. Spread sugar-free pizza sauce on the crust.

3. Sprinkle shredded mozzarella cheese and add toppings of choice.

4. Bake until the cheese is melted and bubbly.

5. Garnish with Italian seasoning and a drizzle of olive oil.

Prep Time: 25 minutes

39. Turkey and Avocado Lettuce Wraps:

Ingredients:

- Turkey slices

- Avocado, sliced

- Lettuce leaves (large, for wrapping)

- Mayonnaise

- Mustard

- Salt and pepper (to taste)

Instructions:

1. Lay lettuce leaves flat.

2. Layer turkey slices and avocado on each leaf.

3. Add mayonnaise, mustard, salt and pepper.

4. Roll up the lettuce leaves to form wraps.

Prep Time: 10 minutes

40. Keto Chicken Caesar Wrap:

Ingredients:

- Grilled chicken breast, sliced

- Romaine lettuce leaves (large, for wrapping)

- Parmesan cheese, grated

- Caesar dressing (low-carb)

- Cherry tomatoes, halved

Instructions:

1. Lay romaine lettuce leaves flat.

2. Add sliced grilled chicken, grated Parmesan cheese and halved cherry tomatoes.

3. Drizzle with low-carb Caesar dressing.

4. Roll up the lettuce leaves to form wraps.

Prep Time: 15 minutes

DINNER

41. Baked Lemon Garlic Butter Salmon:

Ingredients

- Salmon fillets

- Lemon, sliced

- Garlic, minced

- Butter, melted

- Fresh parsley, chopped

- Salt and pepper (to taste)

Instructions:

1. Preheat the oven to 375°F (190°C).

2. Place salmon fillets on a baking sheet.

3. Mix melted butter, minced garlic and chopped parsley.

4. Drizzle the butter mixture over the salmon.

5. Place lemon slices on top.

6. Bake until the salmon is cooked through.

7. Season with salt and pepper before serving.

Prep Time: 20 minutes

42. Keto Beef and Broccoli Stir-Fry:

Ingredients:

- Beef sirloin, thinly sliced

- Broccoli florets

- Soy sauce (low-sodium)

- Sesame oil

- Garlic, minced

- Ginger, grated

- Xanthan gum (optional, as a thickener)

- Sesame seeds (for garnish)

- Green onions, sliced (for garnish)

Instructions:

1. In a wok or skillet, stir-fry sliced beef until browned.

2. Add broccoli, minced garlic and grated ginger.

3. Pour in low-sodium soy sauce and sesame oil.

4. Optional: Use xanthan gum to thicken the sauce.

5. Garnish with sesame seeds and sliced green onions.

Prep Time: 25 minutes

43. Cauliflower Mac and Cheese:

Ingredients:

- Cauliflower florets

- Heavy cream

- Cream cheese

- Sharp cheddar cheese, shredded

- Parmesan cheese, grated

- Garlic powder

- Mustard powder

- Salt and pepper (to taste)

Instructions:

1. Steam or boil cauliflower until tender.

2. In a saucepan, heat heavy cream and cream cheese until melted.

3. Stir in shredded cheddar and grated Parmesan until smooth.

4. Add garlic powder, mustard powder, salt and pepper.

5. Combine the sauce with cauliflower.

Prep Time: 20 minutes

44. Garlic Butter Shrimp Scampi:

Ingredients:

- Shrimp, peeled and deveined

- Butter

- Olive oil

- Garlic, minced

- White wine (optional)

- Lemon juice

- Fresh parsley, chopped

- Salt and pepper (to taste)

- Zucchini noodles (optional, for serving)

Instructions:

1. In a pan, melt butter with olive oil.

2. Add minced garlic and sauté until fragrant.

3. Add shrimp and cook until pink.

4. Pour in white wine (if using) and lemon juice.

5. Season with salt and pepper.

6. Garnish with chopped fresh parsley.

7. Serve over zucchini noodles if desired.

Prep Time: 15 minutes

45. Chicken Alfredo Zucchini Noodles:

Ingredients:

- Chicken breast, cooked and sliced

- Zucchini noodles (zoodles)

- Heavy cream

- Parmesan cheese, grated

- Butter

- Garlic, minced

- Nutmeg (optional)

- Salt and pepper (to taste)

Instructions:

1. In a pan, melt butter and sauté minced garlic.

2. Add heavy cream and grated Parmesan, stirring until creamy.

3. Add cooked and sliced chicken.

4. Season with nutmeg (optional), salt and pepper.

5. Serve the Alfredo sauce over zucchini noodles.

Prep Time: 20 minutes

46. Grilled Steak with Garlic Butter:

Ingredients:

- Steak (your preferred cut)

- Butter, melted

- Garlic, minced

- Fresh rosemary, chopped

- Salt and pepper (to taste)

Instructions:

1. Preheat the grill to medium-high heat.

2. Season the steak with salt and pepper.

3. Grill the steak to your preferred doneness.

4. Mix melted butter, minced garlic and chopped rosemary.

5. Brush the garlic butter mixture over the grilled steak.

Prep Time: Varies based on steak thickness and grilling preferences.

47. Keto Meatball Casserole:

Ingredients:

- Keto-friendly meatballs

- Marinara sauce (low-carb)

- Mozzarella cheese, shredded

- Parmesan cheese, grated

- Fresh basil, chopped

- Olive oil

Instructions:

1. Preheat the oven to 375°F (190°C).

2. Arrange keto-friendly meatballs in a baking dish.

3. Pour low-carb marinara sauce over the meatballs.

4. Sprinkle with shredded mozzarella and grated Parmesan.

5. Drizzle with olive oil.

6. Bake until the cheese is melted and bubbly.

7. Garnish with chopped fresh basil.

Prep Time: 25 minutes

48. Spinach and Feta Stuffed Chicken Breast:

Ingredients:

- Chicken breast, boneless and skinless

- Fresh spinach leaves

- Feta cheese, crumbled

- Garlic, minced

- Olive oil

- Lemon juice

- Salt and pepper (to taste)

Instructions:

1. Preheat the oven to 375°F (190°C).

2. Butterfly the chicken breast.

3. In a bowl, mix fresh spinach, crumbled feta, minced garlic, olive oil and lemon juice.

4. Stuff the spinach and feta mixture into the chicken breast.

5. Season with salt and pepper.

6. Bake until the chicken is cooked through.

Prep Time: 30 minutes

49. Keto Spaghetti Bolognese:

Ingredients:

- Ground beef

- Tomato sauce (low-carb)

- Onion, finely chopped

- Garlic, minced

- Italian seasoning

- Zucchini noodles (zoodles)

- Parmesan cheese, grated

- Fresh basil, chopped (for garnish)

Instructions:

1. In a skillet, brown ground beef with chopped onion and minced garlic.

2. Add low-carb tomato sauce and Italian seasoning.

3. Simmer until the sauce thickens.

4. Serve over zucchini noodles.

5. Garnish with grated Parmesan and chopped fresh basil.

Prep Time: 25 minutes

50. Cauliflower Crust BBQ Chicken Pizza:

Ingredients:

- Cauliflower crust (pre-made or homemade)

- Cooked chicken, shredded

- Sugar-free BBQ sauce

- Red onion, thinly sliced

- Mozzarella cheese, shredded

- Cilantro, chopped (for garnish)

Instructions:

1. Preheat the oven according to the cauliflower crust instructions.

2. Spread sugar-free BBQ sauce on the crust.

3. Add shredded cooked chicken and sliced red onion.

4. Sprinkle with shredded mozzarella.

5. Bake until the cheese is melted and bubbly.

6. Garnish with chopped cilantro.

Prep Time: 25 minutes

51. Lemon Herb Roasted Chicken Thighs:

Ingredients:

- Chicken thighs

- Lemon, sliced

- Fresh herbs (rosemary, thyme, or parsley)

- Garlic, minced

- Olive oil

- Salt and pepper (to taste)

Instructions:

1. Preheat the oven to 400°F (200°C).

2. Place chicken thighs in a baking dish.

3. Drizzle with olive oil, sprinkle minced garlic and season with salt and pepper.

4. Lay lemon slices and fresh herbs on top.

5. Roast in the oven until the chicken is golden and cooked through.

Prep Time: 30 minutes

52. Zucchini Lasagna:

Ingredients:

- Zucchini, thinly sliced lengthwise

- Ground beef or turkey

- Low-carb marinara sauce

- Ricotta cheese

- Mozzarella cheese, shredded

- Parmesan cheese, grated

- Italian seasoning

- Garlic powder

- Salt and pepper (to taste)

Instructions:

1. Preheat the oven to 375°F (190°C).

2. In a skillet, brown ground beef or turkey and season with Italian seasoning, garlic powder, salt and pepper.

3. Layer zucchini slices, meat sauce, ricotta and shredded mozzarella in a baking dish.

4. Repeat the layers and top with grated Parmesan.

5. Bake until the cheese is melted and bubbly.

Prep Time: 40 minutes

53. Keto Butter Chicken:

Ingredients:

- Chicken thighs or breast, cut into pieces

- Butter chicken sauce (low-carb)

- Heavy cream

- Garlic, minced

- Ginger, grated

- Garam masala

- Cumin

- Salt and pepper (to taste)

- Fresh cilantro (for garnish)

Instructions:

1. In a skillet, cook chicken pieces until browned.

2. Add minced garlic and grated ginger.

3. Pour in butter chicken sauce, heavy cream and spices.

4. Simmer until the chicken is cooked through.

5. Garnish with fresh cilantro.

Prep Time: 30 minutes

54. Grilled Asparagus and Parmesan:

Ingredients:

- Fresh asparagus spears

- Olive oil

- Garlic, minced

- Parmesan cheese, grated

- Lemon zest

- Salt and pepper (to taste)

Instructions:

1. Preheat the grill to medium-high heat.

2. Toss asparagus with olive oil and minced garlic.

3. Grill until asparagus is tender and slightly charred.

4. Sprinkle with grated Parmesan and lemon zest.

5. Season with salt and pepper before serving.

Prep Time: 15 minutes

55. Bacon-Wrapped Jalapeño Poppers:

Ingredients:

- Jalapeño peppers, halved and seeds removed

- Cream cheese

- Cheddar cheese, shredded

- Bacon strips

Instructions:

1. Preheat the oven to 375°F (190°C).

2. Mix cream cheese and shredded cheddar.

3. Fill jalapeño halves with the cheese mixture.

4. Wrap each jalapeño with a bacon strip.

5. Bake until bacon is crispy and jalapeños are tender.

Prep Time: 25 minutes

56. Eggplant Parmesan:

Ingredients:

- Eggplant, sliced

- Marinara sauce (low-carb)

- Mozzarella cheese, shredded

- Parmesan cheese, grated

- Eggs, beaten

- Almond flour (or other low-carb flour)

- Italian seasoning

- Olive oil

- Salt and pepper (to taste)

Instructions:

1. Preheat the oven to 375°F (190°C).

2. Dip eggplant slices in beaten eggs, then coat with almond flour mixed with Italian seasoning.

3. Pan-fry until golden on both sides.

4. Layer marinara sauce, fried eggplant and cheeses in a baking dish.

5. Bake until the cheese is melted and bubbly.

Prep Time: 40 minutes

57. Avocado Lime Grilled Chicken:

Ingredients:

- Chicken breasts

- Avocado, mashed

- Lime juice

- Garlic, minced

- Cumin

- Paprika

- Salt and pepper (to taste)

- Fresh cilantro (for garnish)

Instructions:

1. In a bowl, mix mashed avocado, lime juice, minced garlic, cumin, paprika, salt and pepper.

2. Marinate chicken breasts in the mixture.

3. Grill until the chicken is cooked through.

4. Garnish with fresh cilantro.

Prep Time: 30 minutes

58. Keto Cauliflower Fried Rice:

Ingredients:

- Cauliflower rice

- Shrimp, cooked and peeled

- Mixed vegetables (e.g., peas, carrots, green onions)

- Eggs, beaten

- Soy sauce (low-sodium)

- Sesame oil

- Garlic powder

- Salt and pepper (to taste)

Instructions:

1. In a large pan, stir-fry cauliflower rice, cooked shrimp, mixed vegetables and beaten eggs.

2. Add soy sauce, sesame oil, garlic powder, salt and pepper.

3. Cook until cauliflower rice is tender.

Prep Time: 25 minutes

59. Caprese Stuffed Portobello Mushrooms:

Ingredients:

- Portobello mushrooms, cleaned and stems removed

- Fresh mozzarella, sliced

- Cherry tomatoes, sliced

- Fresh basil leaves

- Balsamic glaze (low-carb)

- Olive oil

- Salt and pepper (to taste)

Instructions:

1. Preheat the oven to 375°F (190°C).

2. Place portobello mushrooms on a baking sheet.

3. Layer with sliced mozzarella, cherry tomatoes and fresh basil.

4. Drizzle with balsamic glaze and olive oil.

5. Season with salt and pepper.

6. Bake until the mushrooms are tender.

Prep Time: 20 minutes

60. Creamy Garlic Parmesan Shrimp:

Ingredients:

- Shrimp, peeled and deveined

- Heavy cream

- Parmesan cheese, grated

- Garlic, minced

- Butter

- Lemon juice

- Fresh parsley, chopped

- Salt and pepper (to taste)

Instructions:

1. In a pan, sauté shrimp in butter and minced garlic.

2. Pour in heavy cream and grated Parmesan.

3. Stir until the sauce thickens.

4. Add lemon juice, chopped fresh parsley, salt and pepper.

5. Serve over zucchini noodles or cauliflower rice.

Prep Time: 20 minutes

Appetizers and Snacks

61. Keto Guacamole with Veggie Sticks:

Ingredients:

- Avocados, mashed

- Tomato, diced

- Onion, finely chopped

- Lime juice

- Garlic, minced

- Salt and pepper (to taste)

- Assorted veggies (cucumber, bell pepper, celery) for dipping

Instructions:

1. In a bowl, combine mashed avocados, diced tomato, finely chopped onion, minced garlic and lime juice.

2. Mix until well combined.

3. Season with salt and pepper.

4. Serve with assorted veggie sticks for dipping.

Prep Time: 15 minutes

62. Buffalo Cauliflower Bites:

Ingredients:

- Cauliflower florets

- Buffalo sauce (sugar-free)

- Almond flour

- Garlic powder

- Paprika

- Butter, melted

- Ranch or blue cheese dressing (for dipping)

Instructions:

1. Preheat the oven to 450°F (230°C).

2. In a bowl, toss cauliflower florets with almond flour, garlic powder, paprika and melted butter.

3. Arrange on a baking sheet and bake until golden.

4. Toss the baked cauliflower in buffalo sauce.

5. Serve with ranch or blue cheese dressing.

Prep Time: 30 minutes

63. Cheese and Pepperoni Bites:

Ingredients:

- Pepperoni slices

- Mozzarella cheese, cut into cubes

- Cherry tomatoes

- Fresh basil leaves

- Toothpicks

Instructions:

1. Skewer a pepperoni slice, mozzarella cube, cherry tomato and basil leaf with a toothpick.

2. Repeat for desired quantity.

3. Arrange on a serving platter.

Prep Time: 15 minutes

64. Bacon-Wrapped Avocado Fries:

Ingredients:

- Avocado, sliced into fries

- Bacon slices

- Toothpicks

- Olive oil

- Salt and pepper (to taste)

Instructions:

1. Wrap each avocado fry with a slice of bacon and secure with a toothpick.

2. Place on a baking sheet.

3. Drizzle with olive oil and season with salt and pepper.

4. Bake until bacon is crispy and avocado is tender.

Prep Time: 25 minutes

65. Keto Spinach Artichoke Dip:

Ingredients:

- Spinach, chopped (fresh or frozen)

- Artichoke hearts, chopped

- Cream cheese, softened

- Mayonnaise

- Sour cream

- Garlic, minced

- Parmesan cheese, grated

- Mozzarella cheese, shredded

- Salt and pepper (to taste)

- Keto-friendly dippers (pork rinds, cucumber slices)

Instructions:

1. Preheat the oven to 375°F (190°C).

2. In a bowl, mix chopped spinach, artichoke hearts, softened cream cheese, mayonnaise, sour cream, minced garlic, Parmesan and mozzarella.

3. Season with salt and pepper.

4. Transfer to a baking dish and bake until bubbly.

5. Serve with keto-friendly dippers.

Prep Time: 30 minutes

66. Jalapeño Cheese Crisps:

Ingredients:

- Jalapeño slices

- Cheddar cheese, shredded

Instructions:

1. Preheat the oven to 400°F (200°C).

2. Place jalapeño slices on a baking sheet.

3. Top each slice with shredded cheddar.

4. Bake until the cheese is melted and edges are crispy.

5. Let cool before serving.

Prep Time: 15 minutes

67. Cucumber Slices with Tzatziki:

Ingredients:

- Cucumber, sliced

- Greek yogurt

- Garlic, minced

- Lemon juice

- Fresh dill, chopped

- Salt and pepper (to taste)

Instructions:

1. In a bowl, mix Greek yogurt, minced garlic, lemon juice, chopped fresh dill, salt and pepper.

2. Refrigerate for at least 30 minutes.

3. Serve tzatziki with cucumber slices.

Prep Time: 15 minutes

68. Zucchini Chips with Parmesan:

Ingredients:

- Zucchini, thinly sliced

- Olive oil

- Parmesan cheese, grated

- Garlic powder

- Paprika

- Salt and pepper (to taste)

Instructions:

1. Preheat the oven to 375°F (190°C).

2. Toss zucchini slices with olive oil, grated Parmesan, garlic powder, paprika, salt and pepper.

3. Arrange on a baking sheet and bake until golden.

Prep Time: 20 minutes

69. Deviled Eggs with Bacon:

Ingredients:

- Hard-boiled eggs, halved

- Mayonnaise

- Dijon mustard

- Bacon, cooked and crumbled

- Paprika (for garnish)

- Chives (for garnish)

Instructions:

1. Remove yolks from hard-boiled eggs and mix with mayonnaise and Dijon mustard.

2. Spoon or pipe the mixture back into egg halves.

3. Top with crumbled bacon, paprika and chives.

Prep Time: 20 minutes

70. Keto Sausage Stuffed Mushrooms:

Ingredients:

- Mushrooms, cleaned and stems removed

- Sausage, cooked and crumbled

- Cream cheese

- Garlic, minced

- Parmesan cheese, grated

- Fresh parsley, chopped (for garnish)

Instructions:

1. Preheat the oven to 375°F (190°C).

2. In a bowl, mix cooked and crumbled sausage, cream cheese, minced garlic and grated Parmesan.

3. Stuff mushrooms with the mixture.

4. Bake until mushrooms are tender.

5. Garnish with chopped fresh parsley.

Prep Time: 25 minutes

SOUPS

71. Creamy Broccoli Cheddar Soup:

Ingredients:

- Broccoli florets

- Chicken or vegetable broth

- Heavy cream

- Cheddar cheese, shredded

- Onion, chopped

- Garlic, minced

- Butter

- Salt and pepper (to taste)

Instructions:

1. In a pot, sauté chopped onion and minced garlic in butter until softened.

2. Add broccoli florets and broth, simmer until broccoli is tender.

3. Blend the soup until smooth.

4. Stir in heavy cream and shredded cheddar until melted.

5. Season with salt and pepper.

Prep Time: 30 minutes

72. Keto Chicken Zoodle Soup:

Ingredients:

- Chicken breasts, cooked and shredded

- Zucchini noodles (zoodles)

- Chicken broth

- Celery, chopped

- Carrots, sliced (in moderation)

- Onion, diced

- Garlic, minced

- Thyme and rosemary (dried or fresh)

- Salt and pepper (to taste)

Instructions:

1. In a pot, sauté diced onion and minced garlic until fragrant.

2. Add chicken broth, shredded chicken, chopped celery, sliced carrots, thyme and rosemary.

3. Simmer until vegetables are tender.

4. Add zucchini noodles and cook until softened.

5. Season with salt and pepper.

Prep Time: 40 minutes

73. Tomato Basil Soup with Heavy Cream:

Ingredients:

- Canned tomatoes (unsweetened)

- Chicken broth

- Heavy cream

- Onion, chopped

- Garlic, minced

- Fresh basil leaves, chopped

- Butter

- Salt and pepper (to taste)

Instructions:

1. In a pot, sauté chopped onion and minced garlic in butter until softened.

2. Add canned tomatoes and chicken broth, bring to a simmer.

3. Blend the soup until smooth.

4. Stir in heavy cream and chopped fresh basil.

5. Season with salt and pepper.

Prep Time: 30 minutes

74. Cauliflower and Bacon Chowder:

Ingredients:

- Cauliflower, chopped

- Bacon, chopped

- Chicken broth

- Heavy cream

- Cheddar cheese, shredded

- Onion, chopped

- Garlic, minced

- Butter

- Salt and pepper (to taste)

Instructions:

1. In a pot, cook chopped bacon until crispy.

2. Remove bacon, leaving some fat in the pot.

3. Sauté chopped onion and minced garlic in bacon fat until softened.

4. Add cauliflower, chicken broth and simmer until cauliflower is tender.

5. Blend the soup until smooth.

6. Stir in heavy cream and shredded cheddar.

7. Season with salt and pepper.

8. Garnish with crispy bacon.

Prep Time: 35 minutes

75. Spinach and Feta Egg Drop Soup:

Ingredients:

- Chicken or vegetable broth

- Spinach leaves

- Eggs, beaten

- Feta cheese, crumbled

- Garlic, minced

- Olive oil

- Lemon juice

- Salt and pepper (to taste)

Instructions:

1. In a pot, sauté minced garlic in olive oil until fragrant.

2. Add broth and bring to a simmer.

3. Gradually pour in beaten eggs, stirring to create ribbons.

4. Add spinach and crumbled feta, cook until spinach wilts.

5. Season with lemon juice, salt and pepper.

Prep Time: 20 minutes

76. Creamy Asparagus Soup:

Ingredients:

- Asparagus spears, chopped

- Chicken or vegetable broth

- Heavy cream

- Onion, chopped

- Garlic, minced

- Butter

- Parmesan cheese, grated

- Salt and pepper (to taste)

Instructions:

1. In a pot, sauté chopped onion and minced garlic in butter until softened.

2. Add asparagus and broth, simmer until asparagus is tender.

3. Blend the soup until smooth.

4. Stir in heavy cream and grated Parmesan.

5. Season with salt and pepper.

Prep Time: 25 minutes

77. Keto Taco Soup:

Ingredients:

- Ground beef

- Chicken broth

- Diced tomatoes (unsweetened)

- Green bell pepper, chopped

- Onion, diced

- Taco seasoning (low-carb)

- Cream cheese

- Avocado, sliced (for garnish)

- Cilantro, chopped (for garnish)

Instructions:

1. In a pot, brown ground beef and drain excess fat.

2. Add diced onion, chopped bell pepper, diced tomatoes, taco seasoning and chicken broth.

3. Simmer until vegetables are tender.

4. Stir in cream cheese until melted.

5. Serve with sliced avocado and chopped cilantro.

Prep Time: 30 minutes

78. Pumpkin and Coconut Soup:

Ingredients:

- Canned pumpkin (unsweetened)

- Coconut milk

- Chicken or vegetable broth

- Onion, chopped

- Garlic, minced

- Ginger, grated

- Curry powder

- Butter

- Salt and pepper (to taste)

Instructions:

1. In a pot, sauté chopped onion, minced garlic and grated ginger in butter until softened.

2. Add canned pumpkin, coconut milk, curry powder and broth.

3. Simmer until flavors meld.

4. Season with salt and pepper.

Prep Time: 25 minutes

79. Chicken and Mushroom Soup:

Ingredients:

- Chicken thighs, cooked and shredded

- Mushrooms, sliced

- Chicken or vegetable broth

- Heavy cream

- Onion, chopped

- Garlic, minced

- Thyme (dried or fresh)

- Butter

- Salt and pepper (to taste)

Instructions:

1. In a pot, sauté chopped onion and minced garlic in butter until softened.

2. Add sliced mushrooms and cook until tender.

3. Pour in broth and bring to a simmer.

4. Stir in shredded chicken, heavy cream and thyme.

5. Season with salt and pepper.

Prep Time: 35 minutes

80. Avocado Gazpacho:

Ingredients:

- Avocado, peeled and diced

- Cucumber, peeled and diced

- Tomato, diced

- Red bell pepper, diced

- Red onion, diced

- Garlic, minced

- Vegetable broth

- Olive oil

- Red wine vinegar

- Cilantro, chopped

- Salt and pepper (to taste)

Instructions:

1. In a blender, combine diced avocado, cucumber, tomato, red bell pepper, red onion and minced garlic.

2. Add vegetable broth, olive oil and red wine vinegar.

3. Blend until smooth.

4. Stir in chopped cilantro.

5. Season with salt and pepper.

Prep Time: 20 minutes

SIDE DISHES

81. Garlic Butter Roasted Brussels Sprouts:

Ingredients:

- Brussels sprouts, halved

- Olive oil

- Garlic, minced

- Butter

- Salt and pepper (to taste)

Instructions:

1. Preheat the oven to 400°F (200°C).

2. Toss halved Brussels sprouts with olive oil, minced garlic, salt and pepper.

3. Roast in the oven until crispy and golden.

4. Drizzle with melted butter before serving.

Prep Time: 25 minutes

82. Cabbage Noodles with Bacon:

Ingredients:

- Cabbage, thinly sliced

- Bacon, chopped

- Onion, sliced

- Garlic, minced

- Olive oil

- Salt and pepper (to taste)

Instructions:

1. In a skillet, cook chopped bacon until crispy.

2. Remove excess fat, leaving some in the skillet.

3. Sauté sliced onion and minced garlic in bacon fat.

4. Add thinly sliced cabbage and cook until tender.

5. Season with salt and pepper.

Prep Time: 20 minutes

83. Cheesy Cauliflower Mash:

Ingredients:

- Cauliflower, cut into florets

- Cream cheese

- Cheddar cheese, shredded

- Garlic, minced

- Butter

- Salt and pepper (to taste)

Instructions:

1. Steam or boil cauliflower until tender.

2. Blend or mash cauliflower with cream cheese, shredded cheddar, minced garlic and butter.

3. Season with salt and pepper.

Prep Time: 20 minutes

84. Keto Coleslaw:

Ingredients:

- Green cabbage, shredded

- Carrots, shredded (in moderation)

- Mayonnaise

- Dijon mustard

- Apple cider vinegar

- Swerve or other keto-friendly sweetener

- Celery seed

- Salt and pepper (to taste)

Instructions:

1. In a bowl, whisk together mayonnaise, Dijon mustard, apple cider vinegar, sweetener, celery seed, salt and pepper.

2. Toss shredded cabbage and carrots in the dressing until well-coated.

3. Refrigerate before serving.

Prep Time: 15 minutes

85. Lemon Garlic Asparagus:

Ingredients:

- Asparagus spears

- Olive oil

- Garlic, minced

- Lemon zest

- Lemon juice

- Salt and pepper (to taste)

Instructions:

1. Preheat the oven to 400°F (200°C).

2. Toss asparagus spears with olive oil, minced garlic, lemon zest, lemon juice, salt and pepper.

3. Roast in the oven until asparagus is tender-crisp.

Prep Time: 15 minutes

86. Zucchini Gratin:

Ingredients:

- Zucchini, sliced

- Heavy cream

- Parmesan cheese, grated

- Garlic, minced

- Thyme (dried or fresh)

- Salt and pepper (to taste)

Instructions:

1. Preheat the oven to 375°F (190°C).

2. Layer sliced zucchini in a baking dish.

3. Mix heavy cream, grated Parmesan, minced garlic, thyme, salt and pepper.

4. Pour over the zucchini.

5. Bake until bubbly and golden.

Prep Time: 30 minutes

87. Creamed Spinach with Parmesan:

Ingredients:

- Fresh spinach leaves

- Heavy cream

- Parmesan cheese, grated

- Garlic, minced

- Butter

- Nutmeg (optional)

- Salt and pepper (to taste)

Instructions:

1. In a skillet, sauté minced garlic in butter until fragrant.

2. Add fresh spinach and cook until wilted.

3. Pour in heavy cream, grated Parmesan and nutmeg (if using).

4. Stir until the sauce thickens.

5. Season with salt and pepper.

Prep Time: 20 minutes

88. Rosemary Roasted Radishes:

Ingredients:

- Radishes, halved or quartered

- Olive oil

- Fresh rosemary, chopped

- Garlic, minced

- Salt and pepper (to taste)

Instructions:

1. Preheat the oven to 400°F (200°C).

2. Toss halved or quartered radishes with olive oil, chopped rosemary, minced garlic, salt and pepper.

3. Roast in the oven until radishes are tender and golden.

Prep Time: 25 minutes

SWEET TREAT

89. Keto Chocolate Avocado Mousse:

Ingredients:

- Avocado, ripe

- Unsweetened cocoa powder

- Almond milk

- Keto-friendly sweetener (e.g., erythritol)

- Vanilla extract

Instructions:

1. Blend ripe avocado, cocoa powder, almond milk, sweetener and vanilla extract until smooth.

2. Adjust sweetness to taste.

3. Refrigerate for at least 2 hours before serving.

Prep Time: 10 minutes

90. Almond Flour Chocolate Chip Cookies:

Ingredients:

- Almond flour

- Butter, softened

- Keto-friendly sweetener

- Egg

- Vanilla extract

- Sugar-free chocolate chips

Instructions:

1. Preheat the oven to 350°F (175°C).

2. In a bowl, mix almond flour, softened butter, sweetener, egg and vanilla extract.

3. Fold in sugar-free chocolate chips.

4. Drop spoonfuls of dough onto a baking sheet.

5. Bake for 10-12 minutes or until edges are golden.

Prep Time: 20 minutes

91. Coconut Flour Lemon Bars:

Ingredients:

- Coconut flour

- Butter, melted

- Keto-friendly sweetener

- Eggs

- Lemon juice and zest

- Baking powder

Instructions:

1. Preheat the oven to 350°F (175°C).

2. Mix coconut flour, melted butter, sweetener, eggs, lemon juice, lemon zest and baking powder.

3. Press the mixture into a baking dish.

4. Bake until the edges are golden.

5. Cool and cut into bars.

Prep Time: 25 minutes

92. Chocolate Peanut Butter Fat Bombs:

Ingredients:

- Cream cheese, softened

- Peanut butter

- Cocoa powder

- Keto-friendly sweetener

- Coconut oil, melted

Instructions:

1. In a bowl, blend softened cream cheese, peanut butter, cocoa powder, sweetener and melted coconut oil.

2. Spoon the mixture into silicone molds or form small balls.

3. Freeze until solid.

4. Store in the freezer.

Prep Time: 15 minutes

93. Keto Berry Cheesecake Bites:

Ingredients:

- Cream cheese, softened

- Keto-friendly sweetener

- Vanilla extract

- Mixed berries (e.g., strawberries, blueberries)

Instructions:

1. In a bowl, mix softened cream cheese, sweetener and vanilla extract until smooth.

2. Spoon the mixture into small serving glasses or bowls.

3. Top with mixed berries.

4. Refrigerate for at least 2 hours before serving.

Prep Time: 15 minutes

94. Vanilla Almond Milk Panna Cotta:

Ingredients:

- Almond milk

- Gelatin

- Keto-friendly sweetener

- Vanilla extract

- Sliced almonds (for garnish)

Instructions:

1. Heat almond milk in a saucepan until warm but not boiling.

2. Dissolve gelatin in a small amount of almond milk, then whisk into the warm almond milk.

3. Add sweetener and vanilla extract, whisk until well combined.

4. Pour the mixture into serving glasses.

5. Refrigerate until set.

6. Garnish with sliced almonds before serving.

Prep Time: 15 minutes (plus chilling time)

Beverages

95. Keto Green Smoothie:

Ingredients:

- Spinach leaves

- Avocado

- Almond milk

- Keto-friendly protein powder

- Chia seeds

- Stevia or other keto-friendly sweetener (optional)

- Ice cubes

Instructions:

1. In a blender, combine spinach leaves, avocado, almond milk, protein powder, chia seeds and sweetener.

2. Blend until smooth.

3. Add ice cubes and blend again until well combined.

Prep Time: 10 minutes

96. Iced Bulletproof Coffee:

Ingredients:

- Coffee, brewed and cooled

- MCT oil or coconut oil

- Grass-fed butter or ghee

- Keto-friendly sweetener (optional)

- Ice cubes

Instructions:

1. Brew coffee and let it cool to room temperature.

2. In a blender, combine cooled coffee, MCT oil or coconut oil, grass-fed butter or ghee and sweetener.

3. Blend until frothy.

4. Pour over ice cubes.

Prep Time: 5 minutes

97. Cucumber Mint Lemonade:

Ingredients:

- Cucumber, sliced

- Fresh mint leaves

- Lemon juice

- Keto-friendly sweetener

- Water

- Ice cubes

Instructions:

1. In a pitcher, combine cucumber slices, fresh mint leaves, lemon juice, sweetener and water.

2. Stir well and refrigerate for at least 1 hour to let flavors infuse.

3. Serve over ice cubes.

Prep Time: 10 minutes (plus chilling time)

98. Keto Hot Chocolate:

Ingredients:

- Unsweetened almond milk

- Unsweetened cocoa powder

- Keto-friendly sweetener

- Vanilla extract

- Heavy cream

- Dark chocolate (optional, for extra richness)

Instructions:

1. In a saucepan, heat almond milk until warm.

2. Whisk in cocoa powder, sweetener and vanilla extract.

3. Stir in heavy cream and dark chocolate (if using).

4. Continue heating until desired temperature.

5. Pour into a mug and enjoy.

Prep Time: 10 minutes

99. Matcha Almond Milk Latte:

Ingredients:

- Matcha powder

- Unsweetened almond milk

- Keto-friendly sweetener

- Hot water

Instructions:

1. In a bowl, whisk matcha powder with a small amount of hot water to create a paste.

2. Heat almond milk until warm.

3. In a cup, combine matcha paste, almond milk and sweetener.

4. Whisk until well mixed.

Prep Time: 5 minutes

100. Ginger Turmeric Golden Milk:

Ingredients:

- Almond milk

- Ground turmeric

- Ground ginger

- Cinnamon

- Keto-friendly sweetener

- Black pepper (enhances turmeric absorption)

- Coconut oil (optional)

Instructions:

1. In a saucepan, heat almond milk until warm.

2. Whisk in turmeric, ginger, cinnamon, sweetener, black pepper and coconut oil (if using).

3. Continue heating until well mixed.

4. Pour into a mug and enjoy.

Prep Time: 10 minutes

CONCLUSION

As we come to the end of our exploration of the Atkins diet and its numerous meals, it's time to consider the transforming potential of adopting a better lifestyle. The Atkins diet, known for its low-carbohydrate approach, has not only given a means of losing weight but also fundamentally altered our relationship with food. In this last chapter, we'll go over the essential points, celebrate the journey's accomplishments and offer advice on how to maintain your newfound heath beyond the pages of this cookbook.

Reflections on the Atkins Diet

Dr. Robert Atkins invented the Atkins diet almost four decades ago and it has evolved from a weight-loss technique to a full lifestyle approach. We realized that healthy eating can be a deliciously flavorful and rewarding experience as we went through 100 unique recipes, each carefully prepared to line with the principles of the Atkins diet. The meals ranged from hearty breakfasts to flavorful dinners and decadent sweet desserts, all while adhering to the core principals of low-carb living.

Important Takeaways

1. Understanding Macronutrients: The Atkins diet emphasizes understanding macronutrients, especially carbs. Individuals can impact their metabolism, increase fat burning and accomplish long-term weight loss by deliberately regulating their carbohydrate, protein and fat intake.

2. Nutritional Variety: Our experience demonstrated the necessity of nutritional variety. The dishes used a wide variety of ingredients to ensure a balance of key nutrients. Each meal was designed to give a well-rounded nutritional profile, with lean proteins, healthy fats and an abundance of colorful veggies.

3. Phase Balancing: The Atkins diet is divided into phases, allowing individuals to gradually reintroduce carbohydrates. This technique promotes a sustainable transition from weight loss to weight maintenance, which promotes long-term success. Each phase has a distinct purpose in promoting metabolic flexibility and general well-being.

4. Satisfying and Delicious Meals:

Contrary to popular belief, the Atkins dishes revealed that rich, satisfying meals are not limited to high-carb options.

The journey through these meals demonstrated the wealth of tasty alternatives within the Atkins framework, from sumptuous cauliflower crust pizzas to creamy garlic parmesan shrimp.

5. Mindful Eating and Enjoyment: The Atkins diet promotes mindful eating by emphasizing the significance of savoring each meal and developing a good relationship with food. This technique goes beyond simply nutrition, transforming meals into pleasurable experiences that contribute to general well-being.

Honoring Achievements

As we celebrate the accomplishments of people who began on this culinary adventure, it is critical to recognize milestones attained beyond the numbers on the scale. Weight loss is undeniably significant, but true success is found in the development of sustainable habits and a comprehensive sense of well-being.

1. Weight Loss and Improved Body Composition: Adopting the Atkins lifestyle resulted in significant weight loss and good improvements in body composition for many people. Strategic carbohydrate restriction resulted in increased fat

burning, which contributed to weight loss and the formation of leaner, more defined physiques.

2. Increased Energy and vigor: Many participants noticed an increase in energy and overall vigor. Individuals experienced sustained energy throughout the day by fuelling the body with nutrient-dense, low-carb diets, minimizing mood changes and increasing their capacity for everyday activities.

3. Increased Mental Clarity: Dietary choices have an impact on cognitive performance and mental clarity that extends beyond the physical environment. Participants reported increased attention, enhanced concentration and mental alertness, demonstrating the link between diet and cognitive well-being.

4. Blood Sugar Levels Stabilized: For those dealing with illnesses such as diabetes or insulin resistance, the Atkins diet was crucial in maintaining blood sugar levels. Individuals improved their blood glucose management by reducing their carbohydrate intake, which contributed to improved overall health.

5. Improved Culinary Skills and Creativity: Trying out new recipes not only improved one's health but also inspired

creativity in the kitchen. Participants expressed a renewed love of cooking, experimenting with tastes and discovering the delight of producing nutritious, delectable meals.

Maintaining the Wellness Wave

As we say goodbye to this cookbook, it's important to remember that the journey to optimal health is an ongoing, dynamic process. Maintaining the momentum generated by the Atkins program entails incorporating important ideas throughout daily life.

1. Continued Nutritional knowledge: Maintain a keen knowledge of your nutritional options. When grocery shopping, dining out, or preparing meals at home, pay attention to the macronutrient balance and the quality of the food. This knowledge encourages a mindful and educated attitude to eating.

2. Culinary Experimentation and Adaptation: Continue to delve into the enormous world of low-carb culinary options. Experiment with new recipes, enjoy seasonal vegetables and tweak old favorites to fit the Atkins diet principles. Culinary exploration brings excitement to the journey while reinforcing a long-term, joyful attitude to healthy eating.

3. Mindful Eating Habits: Beyond the scheduled phases of the Atkins diet, cultivate mindful eating techniques. Pay attention to hunger and satiety cues, relish each meal's flavors and cultivate a pleasant and fulfilling connection with food. Mindful eating transforms meals into nourishing rituals that go beyond just nutrition.

4. Regular Physical Activity: In addition to the food part of the Atkins lifestyle, regular physical activity is recommended. Incorporate a variety of cardiovascular, strength and flexibility workouts into your routine. Physical activity not only helps with weight management, but it also improves cardiovascular health and well-being.

5. Social Support and Community Engagement: Get involved in communities or support networks that are dedicated to healthy living. Social support, whether through online forums, local groups, or interactions with friends and family, is critical in maintaining motivation and establishing a feeling of community around similar wellness goals.

As we come to the end of our gastronomic journey through the world of the Atkins diet, let us celebrate our accomplishments, accept the lessons learned and go forward with a renewed commitment to personal well-being. The path to good health is complex and the ideas stated in this cookbook serve as a guidepost for navigating the perilous terrain of nutrition and lifestyle choices.

Each meal is a brushstroke in the magnificent tapestry of life, contributing to the bright portrayal of our health and vigor. May the recipes on these pages continue to inspire, nourish and encourage you as you strive to be a better, more vibrant version of yourself. As you appreciate the flavors of each dish, keep in mind that the route to wellness is a never-ending, ever-changing adventure—a journey worth remembering.

On your ongoing wellness journey, I wish you great health, joy and contentment.

30-Day Atkins Diet Meal Plan

Day 1:

- Breakfast: Keto Bacon and Egg Cups

- Lunch: Chicken Caesar Salad with Avocado

- Dinner: Baked Lemon Garlic Butter Salmon

- Snack: Keto Chocolate Avocado Mousse

Day 2:

- Breakfast: Spinach and Feta Omelet

- Lunch: Turkey and Cheese Lettuce Wraps

- Dinner: Keto Beef and Broccoli Stir-Fry

- Snack: Almond Flour Chocolate Chip Cookies

Day 3:

- Breakfast: Almond Flour Pancakes

- Lunch: Caprese Salad Skewers

- Dinner: Cauliflower Mac and Cheese

- Snack: Keto Berry Cheesecake Bites

Day 4:

- Breakfast: Avocado and Bacon Breakfast Wrap

- Lunch: Keto Cobb Salad

- Dinner: Garlic Butter Shrimp Scampi

- Snack: Chocolate Peanut Butter Fat Bombs

Day 5:

- Breakfast: Keto Chia Seed Pudding

- Lunch: Keto BLT Salad

- Dinner: Zucchini and Cheese Frittata

- Snack: Iced Bulletproof Coffee

Day 6:

- Breakfast: Smoked Salmon and Cream Cheese Roll-ups

- Lunch: Avocado Tuna Salad

- Dinner: Grilled Steak with Garlic Butter

- Snack: Coconut Flour Lemon Bars

Day 7:

- Breakfast: Sausage and Veggie Breakfast Casserole

- Lunch: Broccoli and Cheddar Soup

- Dinner: Lemon Herb Roasted Chicken Thighs

- Snack: Keto Hot Chocolate

Day 8:

- Breakfast: Low-Carb Breakfast Burrito Bowl

- Lunch: Keto Egg Salad Lettuce Wraps

- Dinner: Cauliflower Crust BBQ Chicken Pizza

- Snack: Keto Green Smoothie

Day 9:

- Breakfast: Greek Yogurt Parfait with Berries

- Lunch: Grilled Chicken Salad with Lemon Vinaigrette

- Dinner: Zoodle Alfredo with Chicken

- Snack: Matcha Almond Milk Latte

Day 10:

- Breakfast: Keto Egg Muffins with Ham and Cheese

- Lunch: Shrimp and Avocado Salad

- Dinner: Keto Guacamole with Veggie Sticks

- Snack: Vanilla Almond Milk Panna Cotta

Day 11:

- Breakfast: Coconut Flour Waffles

- Lunch: Keto Chicken Club Lettuce Wrap

- Dinner: Keto Butter Chicken

- Snack: Cucumber Mint Lemonade

Day 12:

- Breakfast: Mushroom and Bacon Egg Bake

- Lunch: Keto Caesar Salad with Grilled Chicken

- Dinner: Cauliflower Fried Rice with Shrimp

- Snack: Ginger Turmeric Golden Milk

Day 13:

- Breakfast: Keto Avocado Toast with Poached Eggs

- Lunch: Keto Chicken Caesar Wrap

- Dinner: Keto Taco Soup

- Snack: Keto Chocolate Avocado Mousse

Day 14:

- Breakfast: Keto Blueberry Muffins

- Lunch: Avocado Chicken Salad

- Dinner: Eggplant Parmesan

- Snack: Almond Flour Chocolate Chip Cookies

Day 15:

- Breakfast: Bacon and Cheese Breakfast Casserole

- Lunch: Keto Sausage and Egg McMuffin

- Dinner: Creamy Garlic Parmesan Shrimp

- Snack: Keto Berry Cheesecake Bites

Day 16:

- Breakfast: Keto Breakfast Pizza

- Lunch: Greek Salad with Grilled Chicken

- Dinner: Lemon Garlic Asparagus

- Snack: Chocolate Peanut Butter Fat Bombs

Day 17:

- Breakfast: Spinach and Mushroom Scramble

- Lunch: Turkey and Avocado Lettuce Wraps

- Dinner: Grilled Asparagus and Parmesan

- Snack: Iced Bulletproof Coffee

Day 18:

- Breakfast: Keto Chia Seed Pudding

- Lunch: Keto BLT Salad

- Dinner: Keto Coleslaw

- Snack: Keto Green Smoothie

Day 19:

- Breakfast: Keto Egg Muffins with Ham and Cheese

- Lunch: Keto Chicken Caesar Wrap

- Dinner: Cauliflower Crust Pizza

- Snack: Coconut Flour Lemon Bars

Day 20:

- Breakfast: Greek Yogurt Parfait with Berries

- Lunch: Shrimp and Avocado Salad

- Dinner: Keto Guacamole with Veggie Sticks

- Snack: Vanilla Almond Milk Panna Cotta

Day 21:

- Breakfast: Spinach and Bacon Salad

- Lunch: Keto Chicken Club Lettuce Wrap

- Dinner: Keto Beef and Broccoli Stir-Fry

- Snack: Matcha Almond Milk Latte

Day 22:

- Breakfast: Almond Butter Smoothie Bowl

- Lunch: Keto Cobb Salad

- Dinner: Garlic Butter Shrimp Scampi

- Snack: Ginger Turmeric Golden Milk

Day 23:

- Breakfast: Keto Chocolate Avocado Mousse

- Lunch: Keto Caesar Salad with Grilled Chicken

- Dinner: Zoodle Alfredo with Chicken

- Snack: Keto Berry Cheesecake Bites

Day 24:

- Breakfast: Bacon-Wrapped Jalapeño Poppers

- Lunch: Avocado Tuna Salad

- Dinner: Cauliflower Fried Rice with Shrimp

- Snack: Coconut Flour Chocolate Chip Cookies

Day 25:

- Breakfast: Keto Blueberry Muffins

- Lunch: Chicken Caesar Salad with Avocado

- Dinner: Keto Taco Soup

- Snack: Keto Hot Chocolate

Day 26:

- Breakfast: Keto Avocado Toast with Poached Eggs

- Lunch: Keto Chicken Caesar Wrap

- Dinner: Grilled Asparagus and Parmesan

- Snack: Iced Bulletproof Coffee

Day 27:

- Breakfast: Keto Sausage and Egg McMuffin

- Lunch: Keto BLT Salad

- Dinner: Eggplant Parmesan

- Snack: Chocolate Peanut Butter Fat Bombs

Day 28:

- Breakfast: Keto Breakfast Pizza

- Lunch: Turkey and Cheese Lettuce Wraps

- Dinner: Creamy Garlic Parmesan Shrimp

- Snack: Keto Green Smoothie

Day 29:

- Breakfast: Keto Chia Seed Pudding

- Lunch: Keto Chicken Caesar Wrap

- Dinner: Lemon Herb Roasted Chicken Thighs

- Snack: Keto Chocolate Avocado Mousse

Day 30:

- Breakfast: Keto Egg Muffins with Ham and Cheese

- Lunch: Shrimp and Avocado Salad

- Dinner: Keto Guacamole with Veggie Sticks

- Snack: Vanilla Almond Milk Panna Cotta

Remember to customize the meal plan based on your preferences, dietary needs and individual responses. Stay hydrated, be mindful of portion sizes and consider any personal adjustments you may need for optimal results. If you have specific health concerns, consult with a healthcare professional or nutritionist.

14-Day Weight Loss Workout Plan

Day 1: Full Body Workout

1. Warm-up: 5-10 minutes of light cardio (jumping jacks, jogging in place)

2. Strength Training:

   - Squats: 3 sets of 12 reps

   - Push-ups: 3 sets of 10 reps

   - Bent-over Rows: 3 sets of 12 reps per arm

3. Cardio: 20 minutes of brisk walking or jogging

Day 2: Cardio Intervals

1. Warm-up: 5-10 minutes of light cardio

2. Interval Training:

   - 30 seconds of high-intensity jogging or jumping jacks

   - 30 seconds of rest (walk in place)

   - Repeat for 20 minutes

3. Cool Down: 5 minutes of stretching

Day 3: Active Recovery

- Engage in low-intensity activities such as walking, yoga, or swimming for 30-45 minutes.

Day 4: Core and Stability

1. Warm-up: 5-10 minutes of light cardio

2. Core Exercises:

   - Planks: 3 sets, hold for 30-60 seconds

   - Russian Twists: 3 sets of 20 reps (10 per side)

   - Bicycle Crunches: 3 sets of 15 reps per side

3. Cardio: 20 minutes of cycling or elliptical training

Day 5: High-Intensity Interval Training (HIIT)

1. Warm-up: 5-10 minutes of light cardio

2. HIIT Workout:

   - Burpees: 3 sets of 15 reps

   - Mountain Climbers: 3 sets of 30 seconds

   - Jump Squats: 3 sets of 15 reps

3. Cardio: 20 minutes of high-intensity cycling or running

Day 6: Rest or Light Activity

Day 7: Long Cardio Session

- Engage in a 45-60 minute brisk walk, jog, or cycle.

Day 8: Full Body Strength

1. Warm-up: 5-10 minutes of light cardio

2. Strength Training:

   - Lunges: 3 sets of 12 reps per leg

   - Chest Press: 3 sets of 12 reps

   - Deadlifts: 3 sets of 10 reps

3. Cardio: 20 minutes of brisk walking or cycling

Day 9: Cardio Intervals

1. Warm-up: 5-10 minutes of light cardio

2. Interval Training:

   - 30 seconds of high-intensity sprints or high knees

   - 30 seconds of rest

   - Repeat for 20 minutes

3. Cool Down: 5 minutes of stretching

Day 10: Active Recovery

Day 11: Core and Stability

1. Warm-up: 5-10 minutes of light cardio

2. Core Exercises:

   - Side Planks: 3 sets, hold for 30 seconds per side

   - Leg Raises: 3 sets of 15 reps

   - Superman: 3 sets of 12 reps

3. Cardio: 20 minutes of cycling or elliptical training

Day 12: HIIT

1. Warm-up: 5-10 minutes of light cardio

2. HIIT Workout:

   - Jumping Lunges: 3 sets of 20 reps

   - Plank Jacks: 3 sets of 30 seconds

   - High Knees: 3 sets of 1 minute

3. Cardio: 20 minutes of high-intensity cycling or running

Day 13: Rest or Light Activity

Day 14: Long Cardio Session

- Engage in a 45-60 minute brisk walk, jog, or cycle.

Remember to stay hydrated, listen to your body and modify exercises as needed. Adjust the intensity based on your fitness level, gradually progressing as you become more comfortable with the workouts.

9 798876 347312